MW01069982

MIND

OVER

MATTER

MIND OVER MATTER

The Uses of Materials in Art, Education and Therapy

DON SEIDEN

Library of Congress Cataloging-in-Publication Data

Seiden, Don.
   Mind over matter : the uses of materials in art, education, and therapy / Don Seiden
     p. cm.
    ISBN 1-890374-02-4 (pbk.)
    1. Art therapy. 2. Artists' materials. I. Title.

RC489.A7 S45 2001
615.8'5156--dc21

                                              2001030294

© 2001 by Magnolia Street Publishers
All rights reserved. No part of this book may be reproduced by any process
whatsoever without the written permission of the copyright holder.

Magnolia Street Publishers
1250 West Victoria
Chicago, IL 60660
U.S.A.

ISBN: 1-890374-02-4
All artwork by Don Seiden
Book and cover design by Sarah Reinken
Printed in the U.S.A.
  2 3 4 5 6 7 8 9 0

Dedicated to my grandchildren...
the minds of our future matter.

Jasmine, Jett, Sam,
Maxie, Kelli, Kim, Jake,
Isabella, Oliver

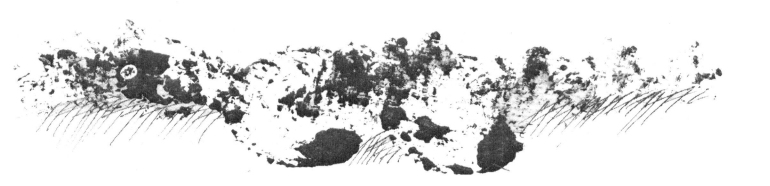

Contents

SECTION II: Experiencing the Elements of Art 59

The Evidence of Experience 101

Mind Over Matter

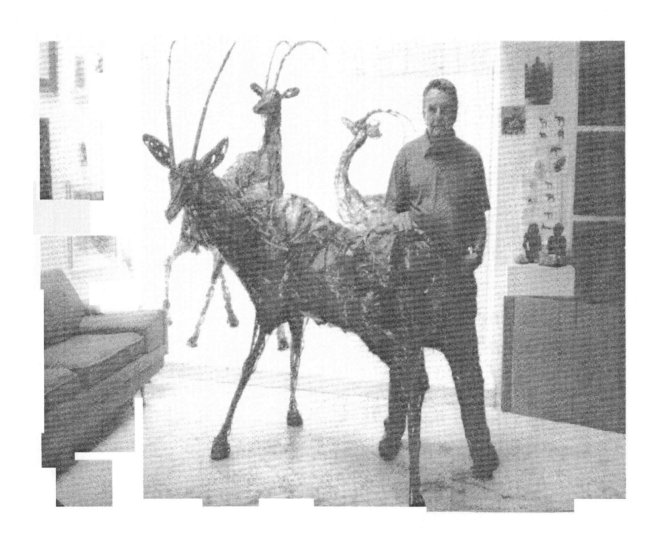

Don Seiden

Introduction

My earliest memories are linked to my senses. I remember an event with a smell. I recall a vision or a taste. I hear sounds and feel textures. These sensory experiences were repeated whenever I made art because the materials that I used tended to stimulate comparable experiences. Materials belonged to the physical world like my own body. When I worked with materials, I envisioned them as having characteristics that reminded me of live things. They were hard and resistant. They were soft and pliable. They were hot or cold, smooth or rough. Later I began to see myself as a partner in the act of creation. The medium and I made art together. We were partners.

When I first became a sculptor I worked with natural materials, stone, clay and wood. I not only experienced the sensory stimulation, but also the feelings of connection to the earth, to the sources. Then came metal. I was able to weld permanent connections, overcome resistance, experience the fire and the chemistry in working with steel, copper and bronze. I fell in love and continue to weld today. Over time I investigated many other materials: paint, drawing materials and printmaking. Then I began mixing methods and materials in my art and I continue to experience the material as an extension of my self.

My art career has crossed many boundaries. I exhibit my sculptures and have taught art in secondary schools, in community programs, and for years in higher education. I have worked in mental health settings and in private practice. I began conducting art therapy when few people in Illinois had heard of it and, eventually, founded the graduate art therapy program at the School of the Art Institute of Chicago. Through it all, I have continued to make art.

My personal history has convinced me that the materials used in art processes are available as bridges toward understanding human connections. This relational approach gives me a better understanding of how the basic elements and principles of art serve as links between artist, object and viewer. I am able to relate to the formal concepts of my art education with a more relaxed and more intimate understanding. Formalism is not too formal after all. People make art and art reflects life.

Don Seiden

Mind Over Matter

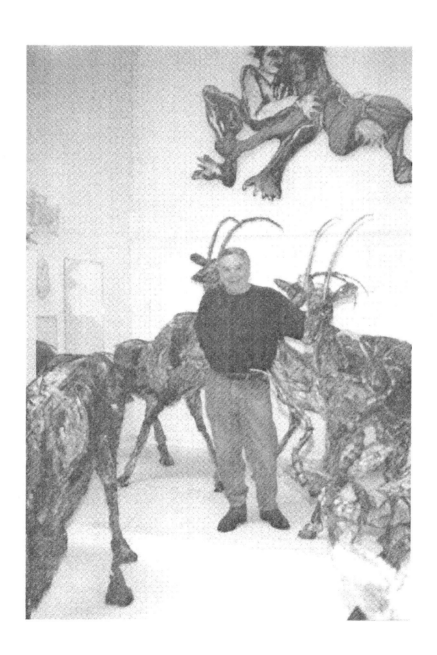

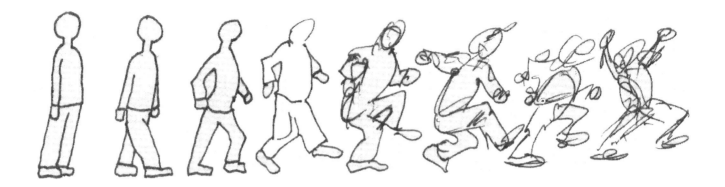

Look Into The Mirror

A full length mirror will reflect your body. A smaller mirror will reflect your face. In both situations you are unable to see your inner organs. You cannot see your mind, your soul, your thoughts and feelings. Yet these invisible qualities are essential elements which define you at least as accurately as your physical being. Your visual perception is limited to that which is visible to the eye. How then do we express what is invisible? Certainly our motion, our gestures, our clothing, our stance and various other expressive modes may be an indication of what we are feeling and thinking to some degree. We read one another's body language. We hear the speech, words and patterns of our human counterparts. We can smell feelings, taste ideas, and see eye to eye. Our sensations are the doorway to understanding one another. Sensations are also the doorway to art expression, and art may very well be the ultimate form of communication because it makes visible the invisible.

Here is a simple experiment. Take a single sheet of plain white paper, such as a sheet of typing paper. The task is to transform this material in any way *without* using a tool other than your hands(body). The limitations are clear. The use of only your hands eliminates your ability to glue, cut or tape, but allows you to experience the many possibilities of your own body as an amazing tool. The hands can tear, crush, roll, fold, and if you want to break rules of gentility, you can stamp on it, chew it, and create a sculpture which expresses any and all of these actions. As you experience your gestures, two things happen: one, the gestures themselves leave a message of what happened—that is, the paper looks as if it was crushed or folded—and two, the object itself begins to take on a life of its own. It has been transformed into an object that conveys the *feelings that were inherent in the actions*. The object carries within it the change of dimension which occurred in the transformation. The object reflects the power of the actions, it *feels* like it was crushed. It may look like something else, a flower, or a twisted rope. The activity has been captured within the object. If you like the object, you can put it upon a pedestal and call it a sculpture. If you don't like it, you can throw it away and simply reflect on the experience and think about what a marvelous thing your body is. The experiment used your whole brain: sensation, motor, memory, emotion, spatial, symbolic and high-level function. If you feel good about this creation, then call it Art. If not, then view it as a experience of self integration. . .body and mind.

Don Seiden

Mind Over Matter

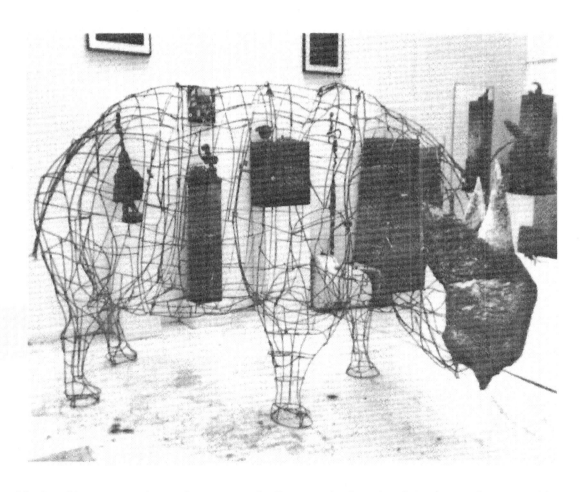

A life-size rhinoceros sculpture in process. The framework of steel rods is ultimately wrapped in heavy aluminum foil and secured with duct tape. Several coats of clear gel medium and acrylic paint weatherize the surface. This piece has been outdoors for about eight years.

Don Seiden

SECTION I: Introduction to Materials

Early in our life experiences we become aware of our bodies. We see, smell, touch, taste and hear our bodies and gradually explore the world of the senses as they define us and the world we inhabit. As humans we are naturally at home in a medium called the atmosphere. We are unable to survive in water or outer space without special equipment. The relationship between the medium and the body is a process which sustains life. Any material that is used for expression or delineation in art is called a medium. A medium can be simply seen as an environment within which matter or substance exists and within which an interactive process is ongoing.

A medium in art making is the environment within which expression occurs, i.e.: paint is the medium within which visual symbols are produced, stone is a medium which is carved into sculpture. Media as substances which carry "messages" are discovered early in life when those objects and things which are familiar develop special characteristics. Toys, blankets, clothes, all merely substances, take on powerful meanings to a child and ultimately throughout life to adults. Our cars, furniture, clothes and other objects carry symbolic value which affect us in significant ways. We are moved in profound ways by the objects with which we live. Political, religious and advertising media utilize the power of materials transformed into symbols as influences to social action. It seems almost like magic or like some supernatural experience when an inanimate object absorbs and then communicates feelings and ideas. How can nonliving matter express living emotion or thought? How is it that children can love a toy and believe that the toy returns the love? How can an artist make images on canvas, paper, wood or stone that are capable of stimulating feelings, thoughts and actions from the viewer?

The art therapist, in approaching materials, must first accept the significance of the nonliving object, matter transformed into some symbolic energy, which is capable of affecting human behavior. "The medium is the message," (a statement popularized by Marshall McLuhan in 1967) implies that the canvas, wood, stone, radio, TV are symbolic messages in themselves. They each have properties which are evocative. The qualities of clay and stone (hard, resistant) or the electronic media (reactive, immediate) all share the power of affecting the human psyche. Add to the inherent properties of media the man made symbols in art, and we can observe a phenomenon which has limitless potential for influence and psychological change.

Certainly the history of materials and tools in art began with readily accessible substances. Humans created objects in stone, clay and wood. They ground pigment from plants and earth and mixed it with blood or urine. The media became more complex as we developed the ability to transform natural material through the intervention of time and physical and chemical processes such as heating natural ore and then creating metal objects. Technology throughout history has expanded to the present both in quantity, variety and certainly quality of art media.

Our attraction and attachment to certain materials is shaped by personal history as well as the enormous influence of culture. All of us have seen, read and heard messages that tell us about "things" that are popular, contemporary and desirable. Our identity is tied to those materials and objects which we choose to own. The things that surround us describe aspects of self which we display to others, or which we hold in private. When we make art we may use some of these cherished materials or find other things from the environment that possess desired attributes relating to our intentions.

If we look to our personal history, each of us has had a natural attraction to certain materials and objects. As artists, we have had experiences with substances that created strong impressions at early ages. Think back to the substances and objects which had power for you as a child. The soft, smooth blanket, the furry toy, the kinetic objects. We all have memories of "things" which seemed almost an extension of ourselves. This idea of object being an extension of self is an important concept in art therapy.

An experiment that may aid in understanding the significance of the early media experiences begins with choosing a material that you experienced as a child: paper, cardboard, clay, mud, sand. Then choose the tools which were also used at that time. Try to attach an age lived to this experience. Were you 4, 7, 9, 12 years old? Try to recapture the quality, style of making things and proceed to make art.

In order to experience the extension of self to objects, choose an object on your person, i.e. a watch, key ring, earring, etc. and describe that object as if it had human qualities. Begin by saying the words, "I am..." and proceed with a description of the object. A strong sense of self definition will emerge as the object is described. These exercises will aid in establishing a base for seeking meaningful connections to the use of materials.

Material Attractors ~ Resistance

In order for materials in art to have effect they must attract or repel us. Some people would love to wallow in a barrel of clay while others feel dirty simply touching the same material. Naturally when working with people in a therapeutic setting the question of materials has to include this range of response. Introducing clients/artists to media when the individuals have no prior experience may involve a natural resistance to the new experience, but particularly a resistance to the use of certain substances. The art therapist can explore the variety of feelings that emerge if he deliberately sets out to work with familiar, unfamiliar, distasteful and attractive media, for the purposes of defining various states of mind and feelings which are stimulated during each of these experiences. When working with individuals, it is important to consider materials which fit the therapeutic goals for the person. It may be important to work with familiar materials, nostalgic materials, new, unusual or even challenging media. In all cases, the directions that the art therapist/educator works toward must include attitudes and symbolic potentials of media. In groups, when the same media is chosen for more than one person, a variety of approaches must be available for meeting individual needs. Painting can be done with tools other than brushes. Hands may be gloved, for example, and many other possibilities explored as well which may satisfy the individual needs within a group.

Conflict/Relatedness

The use of materials together can define relatedness. When crayon and watercolor are used together on the same surface, the crayon "resists" the watercolor and interesting images are formed. The human experiences of harmony, conflict, attraction, repelling and other phenomena are symbolized in our uses of materials when they are brought together in art.

What happens when you bring soft and hard objects together? Opposing colors? Rough and smooth objects? Make art by purposefully connecting oppositions and assess the results. Try to create harmonious groups with a variety of objects. What are the characteristics shared or not shared by certain materials? These are questions which, when answered by artmaking, can aid in helping people to resolve differences in their human relationships as well as defining goals. The use of materials as a symbol of human interaction is a valid form of experimentation that is non-invasive and nonthreatening but one that has metaphoric influence on human behavior.

Transformation

The process of changing from one state of being to another is exemplified in therapy when an individual moves from confusion to order, from inactivity to activity, dysfunction to function or from a disturbed to a more peaceful level of living. This transformation, which often occurs over time, may sometimes be reached more dramatically by sudden insights, medications, and/or vivid experiences. The concept of transformation implies changes in form. The equivalence in art occurs through the creative process. The word creative suggests that something new is emerging from the union of forces that are often in opposition. The union of male and female produce a new human being. It is often an enlightening experience to literally destroy an object and then put the pieces together in new ways. As an exercise in change, one can fragment or take apart something and then rebuild the form. Novel ideas emerge. Transformation is inherent in art, therapy and in life and materials can serve as examples of this experience.

Don Seiden

Mind Over Matter

Don Seiden

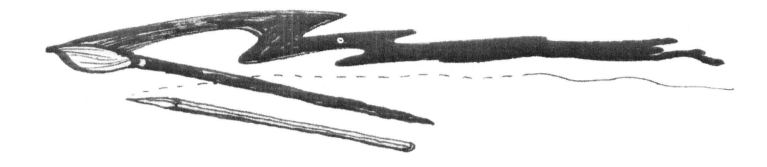

MATERIALS, TOOLS, METHODS

This section is an attempt to explore and personify the identities of various common materials used in art therapy. In order to clarify the nature of any relationship between or among separate entities, human or nonhuman, the differences and similarities of the participating forms must be recognized. The individual characteristics of each party in a relationship can then be seen as related to one another. The mingling and mixing of the characteristics of these participants occur in various patterns yet result in a new form that has qualities of each party present, but is a unique and separate phenomenon. The relationship yields more than the total of its participants.

Materials and tools are described as if they have human characteristics, as if they possess qualities that are as individual and unique as they are in people. Materials and tools are characterized as exhibiting identity, owning a "self", and thus being capable of entering a relationship with another "self" either with the artist or with some other material or tool. These interactions possess symbolic as well as physical characteristics and will be described as exhibiting a variety of relational forms.

These connections can reflect unity, conflict and all the potentials that are available to two or more entities in relationships.

In human relationships, some of the most powerful forms of contact are physical. We are profoundly moved by touch in a variety of forms: loving, sexual, violent, and all the subtleties of these connections. In the making of art, our tactile and visual senses are aroused in symbolic ways by the actual physical contact of instrument to surface, and this contact is similar to human relational experiences. Many of the simple tools of art making can be seen as assertive or aggressive symbols in a simple physical sense. Pencils, brushes, crayons, chalk, knives, chisels and other tools are used to contact a receptive surface or material. The receiving material can be described as receptive in that it receives the instrument, and the relationship which follows is in some ways similar to a human relationship which begins with physical contact and, like art, can develop deeper and more abstract qualities. The instrument and the material influence one another and their relationship becomes as simple or complex as the artist is capable of expressing.

In human physical contact, the effects touch has on our emotions begins at the surface. A fly which lights on the skin's surface will arouse a reflex action accompanied by slight emotional discomfort. The hand of another human on our skin is capable of arousing pleasant or un-pleasant feelings ranging from ecstasy to pain. Visual art such as paint-ing, drawing, sculpture and other related expressive forms are capable of evoking the same range of emotion through symbolic form. The physical contact which is represented by the union of tool and surface, for example, will express the sensitive nature of that contact. The intent, control, impulse and will of the artist determines the ultimate significance of the art. Art therapy begins with basic tools and materials within their own physical context that are guided by the artist to some consummation. In this sense, the artist/client, by creating symbols and relationships, can often attain a feeling of power and mastery which may be an important step toward the recovery of health and strength.

Mind Over Matter

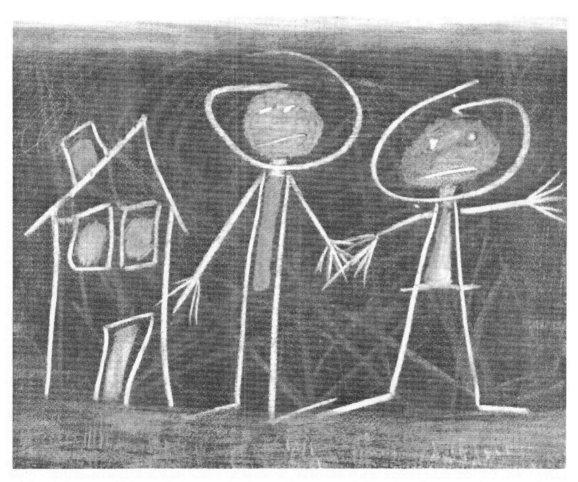

15" x 22" — Scribble, spill, draw and paint as if I were a child. One of a series that stimulated old memories.

Don Seiden

Drawing

media and tools

Many adults who have not experienced artmaking since childhood tend to draw, paint and sculpt as if they are somewhere between the ages of four years through adolescence. The images which they express in art therapy are personal and generally honest attempts to communicate inner thoughts, feelings and fantasy. The ability and skills needed to communicate through imagery may be at a childlike, naive level, yet their expressions derive from the profound life experiences of adults. This gap is sometimes bridged through the use of simple tools and materials that are reminiscent of childhood, and techniques that are familiar and manageable. The relationship between artist and medium can begin in a simple, nonthreatening manner. The artist is inexperienced and naive, the material is ordinary, undemanding and inexpensive. The challenge of materials equals the skill level of the artist. The artist leaves his mark, his personal imagery, through the medium. The medium reflects the artist's experience and thus is no longer ordinary. It now has a unique identity which expresses the will of the artist. The artist also has the potential to be richer for the experience if the relationship with media is pleasurable, interesting, useful or practical in some way. This relationship can be compared to human relationships, and in art therapy friendship, love and pleasure are stressed rather than work or achievement. Ideally, the artist and the material will reflect the nature of their intimacy in a descriptive way.

description of materials

In order to understand the potential of a relationship between artist and medium it is important to know something about both. The unique personality of each artist is expressed through a variety of possible materials, each with it's own special character. The following list describes common materials and tools used in art therapy sessions.

paper

Paper is fragile. It can be torn, cut, burned, crushed and otherwise easily transformed. Paper can be attractive, plain, colorful and tactile. Paper is flat. It can be manipulated by folding, rolling, bending and otherwise changing it into a dimensional object, but in drawing the artist will alter only the surface of paper and the result of this alteration will be a two-dimensional image. The blank surface of the paper is framed by the outer edges, usually a rectangle, square or circle. These geometric shapes represent very secure and clear boundaries. The blankness of the surface, however, can simulate an illusion of vast, empty space. The naive artist is frequently unable to contemplate this "depth" and is limited to relating to the paper as a surface. A surface relationship, however, can be revealing, interesting and seductive in a sensory way. If a depth relationship occurs, it would imply a willingness to take risk on the part of the artist. For the novice to achieve a sense of three dimension on a flat surface may be similar to the sense of fear and adventure which could accompany a beginning swimmer's first entry into deep water. Paper is responsive, vulnerable and open to change. It can be transformed from an ordinary material into a rich and beautiful object, or it can be used and thrown away. It is passive and receptive to manipulation.

other drawing surfaces

Any surface will accept some form of mark or alteration. Surfaces are generally passive, receptive and, with proper instruments, easily altered. Some surfaces are more receptive to certain changes and less to others. Each surface has its own preferences. Even a living surface like human skin can be tattooed. Water surfaces can be changed with oil swirls. Sand, mud and dirt can be drawn upon with a variety of instruments. Some surfaces will absorb liquids, some will repel them. Surfaces can be cut into or built up. Each plane will respond differently to different drawing instruments and will reflect the gesture, the attitude and the character of both the artist and the tool. Exteriors are smooth, slick, wet or dry, rough, abrasive, bland or colorful. The surface of a dimensional form is either representative of what lies underneath or it can be totally unlike its basic composition. For example, a wooden table may have a plastic cover. The clothing which we wear covers our true surface, our skin. A flat surface, a two-dimensional material like paper or cloth, has no three dimensional forms which support it. The flat surface, however, may be altered by a drawing to suggest more dimensional space than it truly has, or the drawing may simply reinforce its true two-dimensional qualities. A drawing should allow the outside to express its own inner qualities and, in fact, may use those qualities as expressive aspects of the image. The union of drawing instrument and surface is an act which can reflect both personalities while creating a third through the image. The artist controls this act of creation by determining the nature of the union and its significance through the image which is left on the surface.

pencil *aggressive*

If paper is passive and accepting of marks, images and manipulation, then the marking instruments can be thought to be aggressive. The instrument touches the surface of the paper and leaves a mark which describes the quality of that union. The mark can describe speed, pressure, width, force and other characteristics which are directed by the artist through the tool and onto the surface.

One of the most common instruments used for marking is the pencil. The graphite pencil is familiar and was used by most people early in life for writing and/or drawing. The pencil leaves a gray mark that can remain permanent or can be erased. The gray color, depending on the softness or hardness of the graphite, lies somewhere between black and white, lighter or darker, but emotionally noncommittal compared to the feeling qualities attributed to most colors. Color pencils are capable of adding these further descriptive qualities but usually not as intensely as paint, for example. Yet a gray pencil mark is still capable of expressing a sensitive range of subtle feelings. The pencil can penetrate, stroke, scribble, record, limit, control, and otherwise effect a variety of symbolic images. The union of pencil and paper can be a profound touch experience or it can be a playful and exploratory activity. The pencil can describe the illusion of depth below the surface and can fill that void with definitive marks or it can skim and move on the surface much like a skater, walker, or runner might move. Try making a variety of gestures while drawing with either hand. The gesture will leave its mark behind the movement on the page. The movement would be recorded exactly as the rhythms and direction occurred. To the naive, untrained and hesitant artist, a graphite pencil is relatively safe. It leaves a mark which can be erased and is not a permanent commitment. It is an ideal tool to stimulate experiment and effect images which range from spontaneous and intimate to cautious and formal. The pencil can be subtle and sensitive to the surface upon which it adheres.

pen

A pen is a powerful instrument. It is similar to the pencil in its aggressive potential but it makes a permanent mark in ink. The image in ink is fixed, cannot be undone without difficulty...it is a commitment. The power of the image is partly in the nature of this attachment to the surface of the receiving material. The pen leaves behind, in its contact, an even, consistent line that is fixed in its dimensions by the size, shape and material of the pen point. The ball-point pen, for example, can roll over a surface. It skates, twirls and leaves a thin but consistent line. The felt-tip pen leaves a range of marks from a fine to broad line. The mark is penetrating and rich in intensity. Color marking pens are nononsense tools. They are decisive, committed, and have a limited but specialized potential for describing their relationship to a surface. The color in the ink is somewhat transparent and the potential for mixing is possible, although generally not in any deep or subtle connection. There are, of course, pens which have more flexibility and potential for variety. These pens can be fitted with a number of different points, each recording a unique character in the line. They are normally dipped into or filled with a finer quality of ink that adds to their sensitivity and range of expression. The use of a pencil can stimulate experimentation, but the pen seems to ask for more certainty and decisiveness from the artist.

color (crayon, chalk, etc.) in drawing

Whereas ink tends to soak into or dye the receiving material, other types of media normally adhere color to surface. The color may be chalk, wax, oil, crayons or other compounds that have mixed characteristics such as the familiar "Cra-pas" which have properties resembling both pastel and crayon. Color added to a drawing complicates the simple relationship between marking instrument and surface. Color is expressive of elusive, personal and hard to define feelings. The colors can be applied in layers, one on top of another or side by side. They can be blended by rubbing or shading. Waxy layers of color can be scratched through using a sharp instrument so that the underneath colors become revealed. Color application using the above instruments in various ways represent relationships with the paper or other surfaces that either flow easily from feeling to form or are more representative of conflicting forces. The color choices and means of relating symbolize feelings of hot, cold, stimulating, relaxing, clashing, flowing, deep or shallow expressions and will, of course, be immensely important in defining the significance of the drawing. The addition of color and the texture left by the drawing tool create a new surface to the drawing; a slick, waxy or oily look, a chalky or dry quality or any other "look" that helps to define the meaning of the image, much like the surface clothing of a person may suggest the above descriptions.

other drawing materials

Any instrument that leaves a mark is a potential drawing tool. Any surface which will accept a mark is a potential drawing. The relationship between the surface and tool is intimate and may represent qualities which are familiar in human relationships ranging between those that produce tension and those that produce relaxation. Seeking instruments and surfaces for drawing can be a stimulating and creative experience. The use of familiar objects in unfamiliar ways or unfamiliar objects in familiar ways are statements about transformation, change and creativity.

Mind Over Matter

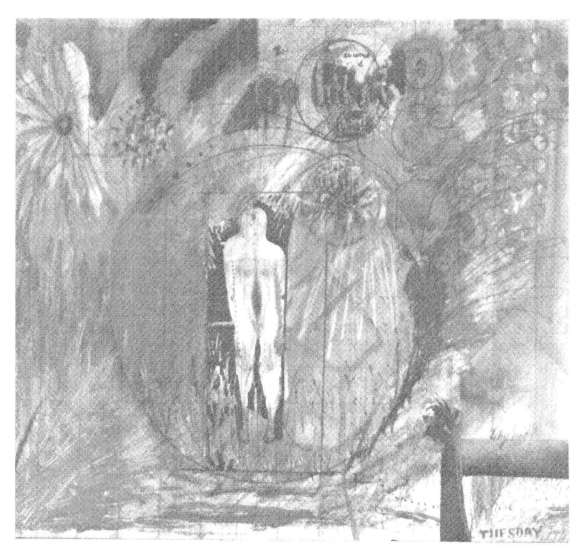

TUESDAY — A painting in acrylic water color that incorporates mixed media: ink, crayon, chalk and writing.

Don Seiden

Painting

paint

Paint is a color-saturated liquid, thin or thick that can be spread over a surface. The pigment is usually a powder which is dissolved in the liquid. Paint can be spread over most surfaces, covering and adhering with a variety of results in the final appearance of the painted surface. Paint will either soak into a receiving surface and color it for as long as the surface remains, or it will stick to the surface for very long periods of time. The surface, being passive, receives the paint and changes itself dramatically. The paint color energizes, floods and charges a surface with feeling as well as with additional significance such as warm or cool qualities, movement forward and backward, as if the color exists in dimensional space or with harmony and conflict.

water color paint

The surface that receives water color is porous. Water is the most basic medium that can be saturated with color pigment.

The surface is generally paper, which was discussed earlier. Water is a natural substance which is essential to life. It is a powerful symbol. Water will easily receive, absorb and saturate to various levels, the color which it receives. The water-saturated color is then transferred to the surface that is then transformed by the imagery the artist creates.

Mind Over Matter

Water color paintings are transparent in that colors and shapes are visible through one another, and the unique intimacy of the relationship between water color and paper is apparent.

oils and acrylics

Color is dissolved in a medium like oil or liquid plastic, both of which are thicker than water. The paint quality of thickness or thinness can vary by adding more or less of another element like turpentine to oil or water to acrylic. When these paints are very thin they behave much like water color, but when they are spread thickly over a surface they tend to change the tactile quality of that surface. Paint can make a smooth surface feel rough or a rough surface smooth with many layers of paint. This quality of density, combined with the greater intensity of color present in its non-thinned state is capable of dramatically redefining the receiving surface. This can be an actual or illusory change in texture. In the relationship between oil or acrylic paint and the surface which is covered, the original appearance of the surface can be profoundly altered so that the receiving material should be chosen more for its structural or functional qualities rather than its appearance. The overwhelming power of this pigment along with the images produced by the artist demand a surface which does not compete with, but rather supports, the final appearance of the painting. To this end, various surfaces offer different qualities like porosity, rigidity, texture, shape, and other characteristics which affect the painting in more subtle ways. The internal dynamics of a painting, the interactions of color, pigment, textures and image combine to create the illusion of life forces that describe the magic of painting.

brushes and knives

Whereas a pen or pencil will normally contact a surface at one point only, a paint brush, palette knife, or any other instrument that is used to spread paint, contacts a wider area. The bristle type, size and shape all affect the way a brush holds paint and the type of mark it makes. A knife or related instrument may be flexible or rigid and must be capable of picking up and spreading paint. The type of tool, its flexibility and shape, determines the appearance of the finished painting. Soft, rough or hard contact will leave a marks that describe the nature of this touch relationship. The choice of instrument, the way paint is applied (i.e. smooth, rough, stippled) and the force, speed, pressure and control that the artist expresses will all effect the feeling and form of the final images.

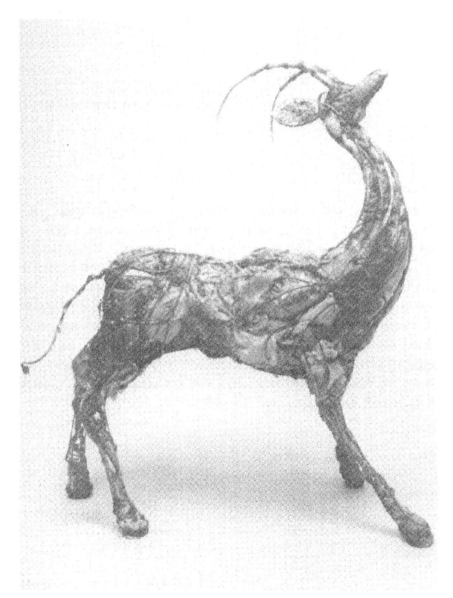

THE FAMILY — One of seven large antelopes. A welded steel and copper skeleton form is "stuffed" with fabric and objects hardened with acrylic medium and painted.

Don Seiden

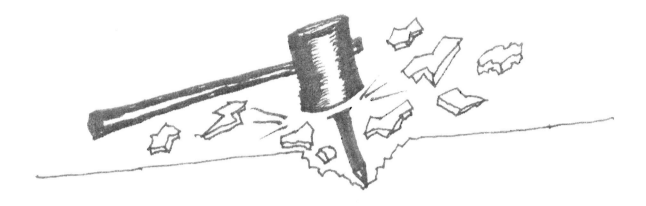

Sculpture

material and tools

Sculpture exists in the round, and possesses three-dimensional qualities of length, breadth and thickness. Mass or volume is a familiar characteristic which is reminiscent of external reality since much physical form which includes human as well as other familiar entities are three-dimensional, exist in space and can be seen from all sides. The feelings which are aroused by a sculpture are often strongly connected to our tactile sense as well as our visual. The relationships which exist between tool and material in sculpture can be more physically dynamic than in the more illusory and abstract considerations of flat or two-dimensional art forms. Space exists around and within a dimensional object and creates both open, penetrating and closed objects. The following section will deal with some of the characteristics of materials and tools that are frequently used in making sculpture with art therapy goals in mind.

clay and modeling

Clay always says "yes." It does not resist manipulation and in fact immediately records and reflects even the most subtle images of touch. From a finger print to poking, pulling, rolling and tearing, clay accepts and records all attempts to transform its shape and surfaces. This malliability, easy availability and enormous versatility makes this medium exceptionally valuable in art therapy. Clay has power in its history, mythology and earth origins which are reflected in its structure. It can be modeled, carved, poured in a liquid state, baked and made rigid. Sculpture of clay can even be constructed section by section. Clay is related in tactile ways to mud, wet sand, and other natural materials including even human feces. This familiarity of touch, accessibility to forming and link with primitive emotions allows the clay sculptor a rare and intimate experience which can range between pleasant to very unpleasant sensations. Clay work can stimulate relaxing, flowing and permissive behavior or it can create confusion and anxiety because of its lack of boundaries and resistance.

Clay particles can be suspended in water or oil and the properties differ. Water-based clay will dry out if not kept damp. Oil-base clay will not dry and can be used indefinitely. Water-based clay can be fired in ovens at high temperatures and will completely change from the plastic and passive state to a rigid, hard and permanent form. Oil clay remains in a plastic state and can never retain a permanent and rigid quality. Clay allows for exploration, testing of limits, subtle to obvious expression and can be worked directly using the hands or indirectly with various tools or implements which leave their marks. Clay is a medium which is open to a variety of relationships the quality of which depend on the desire and gesture of the artist and the nature of the material. Clay, as well as other modeling materials have physical growth potential. These substances may also be described as "additive" since they expand in size through the addition of material to the mass. Portions of clay can be also be removed or shifted to another area of the piece. Any substance that exists between a liquid and a rigid state and has a degree of thickness, retains a shape, and can be affected by manipulation can be used as a modeling material.

other modeling materials

Familiar substances like dough, paper mache, cloth dipped in plaster, putty, modelling pastes, and even gauze impregnated with the type of plaster used in hospitals to make plaster casts for broken bones are available for sculpture. Of course, the identity and nature of each of these materials is somewhat different from one another and their response to the touch of the artist will vary as well as their final appearance. But they all share the plasticity of materials which can be modeled. They are accepting of change, nonresistant when wet and reflective of spontaneous as well as labored expressions. They personify qualities of behavior which reflect human passivity, submission, ease of change, flow, nonresistance, reflectivity and acceptance. These qualities allow the artist to express his or her power, create energy and a sense of control that is an especially valuable experience in art therapy. The artist in a relationship with a nonresistant material is able to overcome his or her feelings of helplessness by acting upon a substance, altering and transforming its nature and by expressing a personal statement through the media.

construction

Materials which are suitable for construction ideally should be rigid and able to support weight. These materials are connected in some fashion and thus are built up or out. They form either structural shapes which are sculptural statements in themselves or skeleton-like shapes which will support a covering "skin" of another material. In art therapy the act of construction may symbolize the building and/or rebuilding of personal goals. Construction is a way of expressing growth, strength to support, dependency, unity, commitment and other values attributed to positive human experience. These characteristics of building are explored in sculptural construction and hopefully are translated into the actual life experience of the client/artist.

The materials that are used in construction are three-dimensional or at least are capable of forming three-dimensional objects. They include paper (rolled, folded and formed), wood (toothpicks, tongue depressors, scraps or found shapes), metal (wire, rods, sheets) and all kinds of found or manufactured objects. Natural materials, such as stone or driftwood, can also be connected to form sculpture.

The importance of attaching separate parts is a key element in construction. Parts of the sculpture are connected and joined in various ways. Nailing, gluing, soldering, welding, folding, clipping and other joining techniques are utilized depending on the nature of the materials to be joined. The joints themselves are either permanent or temporary and express characteristics which define the nature of joining. Joints are places where separate things come together and thus become symbols of relating which are described by these connections. Construction is risky because each joined part can be a weak area if not carefully brought together and so demands some perseverance, attention to detail, problem solving skills and care from the artist. But heights can be reached, control exhibited and the fulfillment and accomplishment in a very concrete form is possible. Knowing the materials and relating them in sensible and appropriate ways is a guarantee of some success in this technique. A knowledgeable art therapist can aid in the decision-making involved in construction.

carving

The process which involves materials that can be carved may be described as "subtractive". The substance which is carved loses material until the final chosen image is all that remains. Removing material to release the inner image generally implies that the medium is resistant to the tool. In fact, although materials like clay or even butter can be carved, we tend to think of carved sculpture as dealing with mass as well as resistant material (i.e.: stone, wood, etc.) and so it is not limited to merely altering surfaces but instead transforming the inner and outer layers of material. In the act of carving, the tools that are used are often abrasive (files, rasps, etc.) and sharp (cutting chisels, picks and knives). They tend to involve energetic and sometimes aggressive movements such as hammering, sawing and penetrating. In art therapy, because of restrictions in use of materials, space and tools, more resistant media is sometimes not available and softer, more passive materials such as soap, plaster, balsa wood, or fine brick are substituted for traditional sculpture media like hard woods or stone.

Carving and its unique relationship between tool and medium is a more aggressive experience than most of the art forms previously discussed. Cutting away and removing material is essentially a destructive act. The fact that creativity arrives out of this "violence" is an experience which allows the artist the unique opportunity to express hostile and angry feelings alongside the loving feelings associated with creating art. Carving represents a relationship that combines opposites and so it can be described in some ways as an act of reconciliation. It is also a battle between an aggressive tool and a resistant material that ideally results in a unity of forms and feelings. The artist benefits from this experience by expressing his power over the medium and by releasing the image from its "prison" of substance. Through this process, the final sculpture can be seen as a symbol of freedom and creativity.

casting and mold making

Casting is a process where a negative space is filled with a liquid that hardens. The positive form is then removed. This, in a simple way, can be described when a slab of clay is pressed in one section and a nega-

[handwritten margin note: a way to release anger]

tive valley is created. The valley is filled with, for example, liquid plaster. The plaster hardens and a shape is removed which reflects the negative shape in reverse. A "hill" is now formed in plaster. Molds can be created from various forms and materials to reproduce shapes either singly or in quantity over and over again. A metaphor can be seen in the statement "he is cast from the same mold as his father".

Mind Over Matter

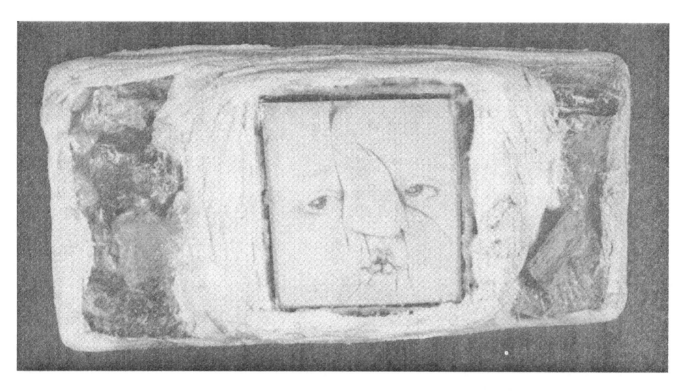

AIRLESS — A stuffed, sewn and crushed face in a plastic box surrounded by a variety of found objects.

Don Seiden

. . . And More
fabrics and fiber

Weaving, knotting, sewing and other methods of working with fiber and fabric may result in objects that combine qualities of dimension. Cloth, for example, is woven and designed as a two- dimensional form, but may ultimately become an article of clothing and thus cover and define a three-dimensional form. Fibers, like yarn, rope and string may be knotted, sewn and frayed to form sculptures, both hanging and even free standing. Images can be sewn, drawn, printed and painted on fabric, and by crushing, folding, tying and dipping into color dyes, free form and spontaneous images can be created. Fabric hardeners may be used to soak cloth which dries into rigid shapes. All these methods can then be combined in various ways.

These materials are familiar to most people, and client artists are able to create interesting and unusual forms with relatively simple skills. Although the final product in fiber and fabric is important in a visual sense, the making of the object involves a strong tactile connection as well. The texture of cloth can be stimulating and even sensual. The texture of yarn or rope can be intimately reminiscent of human hair. Weaving, sewing and tying are activities which stress integration so that these experiences symbolize the coming together which results in unity. Working with fiber and fabric, particularly for people who are fragmented and confused, can be a most satisfying activity. It can be sensual, integrating, and may also result in the making of practical as well as aesthetically pleasing objects.

The materials used in these activities share certain physical qualities. They are soft, flexible, fibrous and when draped over a solid form they follow its general contours. These materials offer little resistance to cutting and shaping. They can be held together in various ways, including sewing, tying and lacing.

mixed media

Scrap, found, fabricated, old, useless, worn, inexpensive, abundant, commonplace objects and the printed image are all potential art materials. A single object may sometimes be chosen for aesthetic reasons by the artist, it can be removed from the flow of life, set apart and described as art. An object may be reshaped, changed in some way, or combined with other objects and be seen as art. This potential for transforming the objects of everyday experience, the ordinary, into the unique or extraordinary is a valuable art therapy concern. These materials are generally preformed but are changed in their new relationship to the artist or to one another. The client/artist is often able to identify with this process of change from the ordinary to the unique. It is a familiar experience for people who themselves feel helpless, useless, worn, old, sick or simply anonymous to wish, like Cinderella, to be transformed into a thing of beauty. This process can be symbolized through the use of found material as art media. The magic of the art experience may be most intensely felt by people using scrap materials in art who might otherwise be intimidated by more traditional media that are often associated with special skills and achievement.

The use of mixed media is an exercise involving sorting, selection, judgment and arrangement. Often, the objects used are not altered but simply chosen and committed to connections with one another or to a surface. The results of mixed media can be two-dimensional (collage, montage) or three-dimensional (sculpture). Three-dimensional objects or flat materials can be attached by various methods ranging from less permanent (paste, glue) to more permanent (screws, nails, soldering or welding). The nature of this attachment represents a need for confidence in making those decisions that represent varying degrees of commitment. For client/artists who exercise their decisiveness, to risk commitment, even symbolically, can be a beneficial experience, especially when guided by a sensitive art therapist. The use of aluminum foil to make basic shapes was further developed by this author when he discovered that the shapes could be taped together and otherwise joined. The tape (preferably duct tape) could then be painted and flexible sculptures created. Many artists will collect things and arrange them in various ways thereby creating *installations* that transform an environment.

printmaking and related techniques

These activities in art therapy involve relatively simple techniques for reproducing and/or transferring images from one material to another. A typical printing procedure involves first creating an image by gouging and removing material from a flat surface such as metal, plaster, linoleum, wood or any material which can be carved in this manner. The material is removed in such a way as to leave raised (uncut) and lowered (material removed) surfaces. Ink is then rolled over this "plate" and the image is then transferred to paper or another surface by applying enough pressure to the imaged substance to allow the ink to adhere to the new surface. Objects such as gum erasers, potatoes or wood scraps can be carved in this way and, like rubber stamps, they can reproduce the same image over and over using ordinary inked stamp pads. Printmaking expresses certain physical characteristics of the material on which the original image is created. For example, a wood-cut will leave traces of wood grain on the print so that even the original experience of creating is reproduced on other surfaces. Printmaking and stamping involve the client/artist in some important activities. The fact that an image is created by literally penetrating, gouging, and scratching and otherwise altering a material is not only a physically expressive act, but one in which an image can be reproduced. The reproduction of an image suggests longevity which in turn can be reassuring to a client/artist who may respond to the repetition as a symbol of continuity.

Many soft surfaces can be scratched into, gouged, or raised, such as linoleum or styrofoam which may be used for printing. Ink can be rolled onto a plastic or glass surface and marks scratched into the ink will leave a negative image. A paper then is placed over the image, pressed and then raised to reveal the printed surface. Power and control over the material and in addition a sense of continuity and confidence in the future are symbolic experiences which the act of reproduction fosters. Stamping is a familiar, repetitive activity that can aid in releasing certain physical tensions.

Another related activity is the making of rubbings. Paper is placed over a surface which possesses interesting textural qualities. Crayon or chalk is then rubbed over the paper. The imprint of the surface is left on the paper. This experience involves the artist in an intimate experience with the surface being rubbed. The tactile quality is enjoyed and the accuracy of the image produced connects the visual sense to the texture. Better sensory integration (visual and tactile) aids the client/ artist in achieving an identification with the "real" world, a sense of rhythm and flow, fresh perceptual experiences and the pleasure of "possessing" the surface which was reproduced.

photography, video , filmmaking and computer graphics

The use of technology in art therapy reduces the need for manual skills in the production of images, but emphasizes instead perceptual and conceptual relationships. The client/artist may need only know how to push a button (as in Polaroid instant photography) to achieve a complete and accurate image. The ease of manipulation focuses attention on the picture itself. What am I seeing? How are elements relating? What does the picture say? These questions present themselves to the artist and the picture itself answers them.

Because film and video are capable of presenting accurate, recognizable images of life activities, still or in motion, the potential for the viewer to identify with these images is present. People are able to see themselves and others in ways that are often revealing and helpful. The environment can be a source of treasure when an image seeker is searching for pictures.

The camera "shoots" a picture. The photographer "captures" an image with the camera. The quality of possession is evident. In a magic way we "possess" the reality when we have a photograph. Motion pictures and videotape adds still other elements to the sense of reality. Movement and sound become additional sense experiences. Computer generated images are another source of power for the client/artist who can manipulate electronic media and, with the click of a mouse, produce astounding results.

The use of these techniques are often limited in art therapy. There are economic, space and many technical drawbacks—even legal restrictions on the use of equipment in certain settings. But creative art therapists have found ways to overcome many of these obstacles and the image making potential of these technologies is enormous.

Don Seiden

Mind Over Matter

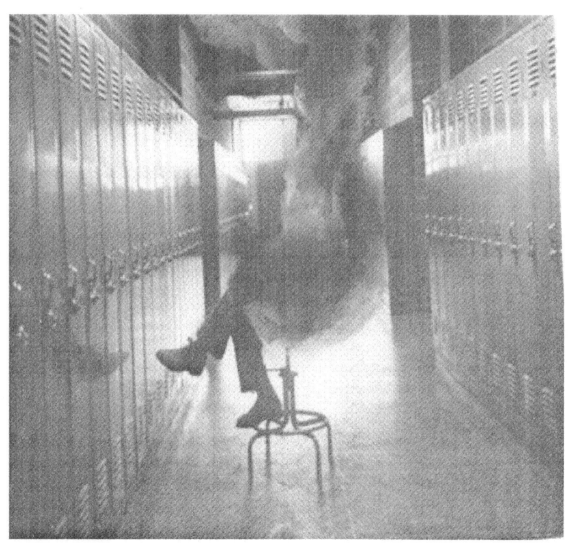

DISAPPEARANCE — The original photo is altered by painting "smoke" then rephotographed and printed.

Don Seiden

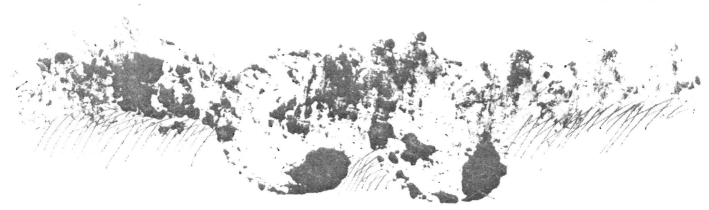

SECTION II: Experiencing the Elements of Art

The previous section dealt with the materials and tools used in making art. This section will attempt to define the elements of art, the visual symbols, the parts which, when combined, make up the whole.

A tool acting upon a material does not act of its own power. The artist exercises the power that guides the physical material and manipulates media until a statement that reflects the relationship between artist, tool and material is created. The finished work of art is a record, a document of the relationship between the artist and his product. The product is a unity, a complete entity made up of abstract elements, symbols, marks, color, line, balance and other aspects of what the artist would call form. Form includes not only these above elements, but also the subject matter or content. The subject matter describes what the work is about. Content makes a statement which can range from personal to universal in scope. The work can be about life, culture, politics, trauma, about art itself or even about the simple movements or gestures of the artist which leave marks as a statement about that relationship.

The attempt to produce art by an artist/client who may be inexperienced in this undertaking, is often an attempt to record images of his inner world. The feelings, fantasies and ideas of the artist must be measured against the limitations of the material, his skills and his experience. These limitations affect the degree of accuracy both in his perception and in his ability to express and communicate that perception. Each medium (drawing, painting, sculpture, etc.) sets its own limits and quality of imaging so the choice of medium should reflect as closely as possible the vision of the artist. Thus, the first decision made by the artist/client is the choice of medium.

Art therapy views the art process as a path to the unconscious, a way of mirroring inner experience as well as a form of release for those perceptions that may be best expressed through art.

The symbols that are combined to produce visual art, for example, may include lines, shapes, textures, color, space and other elements that together make up an image that defines the artist's perceptions of the world.

We will attempt to describe and relate those elements to the artist's motivation and to their origin via the physical contacts of media and tool. These various basic elements can all be expressed through any medium. Line and color, for example, may be expressed in painting, drawing, sculpture or in any other medium. The communicative potential of each of the separate elements is enormous. Together they create the complexity of art's symbolic power.

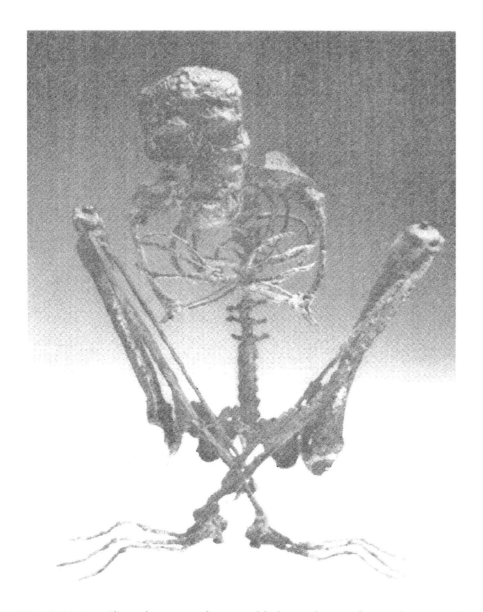

LIZARD WOMAN — Silicon bronze rods are welded together to form a linear sculpture.

Don Seiden

Line

A line is the interface between two forms. It divides, separates and connects. A line has a starting point and proceeds in any manner of direction, curves or angles, to arrive at another point. It can be open ended or it can describe the contours of a shape and reach its conclusion back at the point of its origin. In nature, when two forms meet one another, the line that is formed is essentially an illusion.

In art therapy it is important to recognize the symbolic content of human expression. Human action is functional in that it leads to attainment of goals, but part of its function is symbolic, that is, the behavior may have meaning that goes beyond its obvious purpose. Every experience is multidimensional. We eat primarily to stay alive, but eating has many additional purposes and meanings such as ritual and pleasure. Work, play, sleep and all human activity has symbolic as well as functional value. In the production of art, the symbolic, metaphorical value of the experience is an essential component in that it allows for the fullest exploration of an idea or feeling. In order to understand this chain of association and its value, let us look at the significance of LINE in art.

In nature, we look out over the lake or ocean where the sky meets the water. The unbroken horizon is a straight horizontal line. It connects and separates. It is peaceful and continuous. We may witness the jagged and abrupt line of lightning in a storm. It is powerful and dangerous. The significance which we attribute to these linear events begins with the information which describes their function, but includes as well, the emotions experienced when we view these phenomena. If asked to draw a horizon line or lightning using a pencil and paper we might simply draw a horizontal line — or a jagged line /\/\/\/. These are symbols which describe the fundamental line qualities of each experience within the limitations of the shape of paper. The line begins in each case with a point. The point of the pencil contacts the paper and is drawn across the page in a chosen direction. The line begins and ends. It describes the movement. It separates forms and connects both sides as an interface. It is familiar, repetitive and directs the viewer's eye across the page. The qualities that a line may reflect visually include speed, intensity, pressure, width, light, darkness, hesitation, confidence, meandering, accuracy, force, purpose, rhythm, unity and innumerable other symbolic and functional characteristics. In a simple line drawing, however, it is often difficult to interpret the subject, the content or theme of the work since the line may mean so many things to so many people. A line across a page could be the horizon, a path, a road, border, incision and on and on. Only the artist may know what specifically is meant by this mark. A jagged line may be lightning, broken glass, cracks in the sidewalk, etc. One goal of the artist is to draw a line so that it contains the qualities which describe, express and communicate the phenomenon being symbolized. The goal of the art therapist is to aid in this process. When straight lines cross one another coming from different directions they create grids, lattices or webs. These forms resemble fields upon which other things may rest as on maps, thus helping us find our way by observing intersections and directions.

Don Seiden

In art therapy one of the primary tasks of the artist/client is to describe his inner world. Feelings and thoughts are expressed visually in an attempt to communicate the unconscious experience as clearly as is possible. The concept of LINE now takes on additional significance that may describe a particular state of being.

To express, in a line or series of lines, the state of being or the feelings of the artist/client may require a spontaneous and gestural approach to line-making. Since feelings are not fixed they may best be described by lines which are drawn without much planning or thought. An impulsive scribble, doodle or mark may more accurately reflect the inner state of the unconscious than will a more determined effort. The potential of the art experience, however, allows for an endless clarification so that the artist may begin by spontaneously drawing lines and end after further refining them in a more purposeful manner. LINES, in their infinite variety may be like individual words in the sense that they are symbols which help to answer the questions, "How do you feel?", "What do you think?".

Mind Over Matter

Saunter - proceed slowly

symmetry - balance, harmony, harmonious arrangement

equivalence, harmonious

Solicitous - Anxious/concerned

expressing care/concern, full of desire

eager

Don Seiden

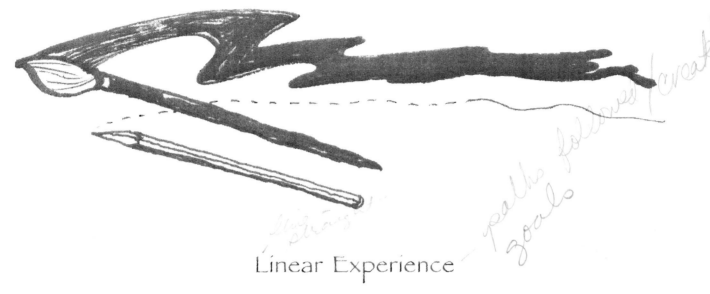

Linear Experience

The manner in which a person moves in a space from one point to another is a linear activity. Some people move in straight lines, that is they perceive a desired target and in direct, functional ways move to reach and attain their goal. Other people may perceive desirable goals but because they tend to be distracted, they meander in irregular patterns and may even ultimately lose sight of their goal. Meandering, however, may be a particularly enjoyable and relaxed experience when goals are not specific or of concern. Paul Klee spoke of "taking a walk with a line." Conversely, people who seem to always know where they are going and always choose the quickest and most expedient method of arriving may also create very rigid patterns which inhibit their behavior and leave the joy of wandering aimlessly to others. Linear behavior in its extremes may create confusion on one hand and inflexibility on the other.

Most life activities are based on our ability to follow the paths or lines that others have created. We walk or drive on walkways and roads. We follow the "beaten path" in order to arrive at conventional goals. Our task is simplified by knowing how others have mapped out our common space and common goals in linear ways. Problems may arise, however, for the individual who is unable or unwilling to follow the lines created by others. The person who is disinclined to pursue the same course as most others must explore unknown territory and create new paths toward unique desires. Exploration may also result in confusion, loss of direction and the sense of self when an individual loses his way and becomes swallowed up in the immense world around him. When we walk along our personal lines or life paths we may look ahead and behind and we see the oneness of the future and past, but the line which we create in our movement divides our right side from our left and thus creates a duality, a division in our present. The line divides space. Our vision of a self, in linear terms, is then partially defined by the duality that we perceive in space. This duality is confirmed in our physical, emotional and intellectual form in many ways, i.e. the bilateral brain, symmetry of the body and awareness of conscious and unconscious forces. When we are still and not moving, our perception tends to emphasize the oneness or unity of nature and the self. When we are in motion we become aware of direction, linear force, and therefore of divided space. The self is, then, both a unity as well as a duality in relation to movement and to the line which it creates. As humans we possess a single, dual and multiple identity simultaneously.

Linear patterns are present not only in external space but within our own bodies. Our blood moves along direct pathways. Our nerves are lines of communication which carry messages from one area to another. Thinking itself is often linear activity which is sequential and follows logical directions. Reading, writing and most goal-oriented activities are linear in form and possess similar characteristics of the line in a drawing, such as speed, pressure, depth, continuity, straightness, curves, etc. Our language contains references which describe linear activity in relation to self, such as "crossing the line," "lining up", "boundary line," "line of talk" and other idiomatic phrases that describe human activity.

In art, the line can be created for many purposes. It can define space and direction. It can be an element that describes shapes and action with feeling as well as function. Art therapy is an experience that may define and design life activity in terms of art elements. The line in a drawing may reflect movement, goal orientation, direction, exploration, relaxation, rigidity and many other qualities that an individual must deal with in his life. The line in art may be changed and altered in form and purpose. It can symbolize the human experience and provide insight and a chance to plan for desired change. The line in art is directly related to the life line.

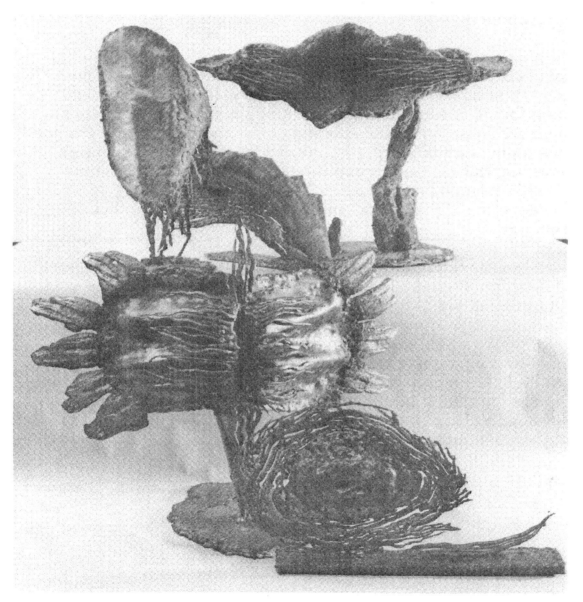

SEAFORMS — A series of sculptures created by fabricating and welding copper sheet and bronze rods.

Don Seiden

control
Cabels

Shape

A shape is defined by its boundaries or edges. It is an entity separate from other entities and it has a unique spatial form. At its limits, the shape meets its environment and interacts with other shapes, other entities. In the preceding section, a line was described as possessing qualities that distinguish it from other lines. When a line intersects with itself on a flat plane, it creates a shape. The shape, then, is out-lined, and it's dimension, limit and general appearance are defined by the line.

When a person is introduced to the concept of shape and becomes aware that the universe, which is shapeless, is filled with elements of many different shapes, it may be useful to identify these different items. One means of identification is by naming familiar shapes. We share and communicate the symbols in words and shapes which iden-tify, for example, circles, squares, triangles and their three-dimensional counterparts in space, the sphere, cube and pyramid. We have histori-cally and culturally passed on additional meanings for these shape symbols which share certain characteristics. There are, of course, an infinite number of shapes which are not easily identified by name or category. There are organic entities that change their shape constantly and there are stable shapes that are so irregular in their appearance that they might be called free-form.

Shapes not only separate themselves from the surrounding space, but they also contain space and/or other shapes as well. This quality adds dimension to the meaning that even the shape communicates. A single shape can tell us something about its function. It can convey information about its strength or weakness and its potential to attract or repel. Shapes, particularly when they are familiar and simplified (for example: the circle, square and triangle), convey meanings which have historical and mythological origins. The unity, continuity and absolute center of a circle may seem to convey qualities of peace, balance and contemplation to the artist and the audience. The square with its angles, corners and straight lines has function in building, dividing space and measuring. It has strong connections to the earth and the practical concerns of living. The triangle, broad-based and to its points, for many people has been representative of organizational hierarchy as well as symbolizing spiritual and secular ambition.

The artist/client gradually may become familiar not only with shapes in the environment that express certain characteristics, but also personal shapes as well, that are based on private inner feelings. Just as an outline encloses space, when rendered in art these shapes may reflect a variety of feelings and thoughts made finite by the act of shaping and by creating boundaries for these otherwise abstract phenomena.

Of all the concepts in art-making, the shaping of media may be the most difficult for the art therapy client. The individual in therapy is a person who is often in "bad shape". The ability to create and understand limits, boundaries, to create an entity which is self-sufficient and able to relate to other shapes is dependent to some degree on how a person views his own external and internal space. If a person feels misshapen in any way, that feeling will influence his perception and ability to form spatial entities. A sensitive art therapist may aid the client/artist in the process of rebuilding, redesigning and recreating strong and significant shapes which may communicate more positive, sturdy statements.

Shape defines the person, the self, in terms of its boundaries and its unity. One of the simplest visual determinations of the identity of a thing is its shape. We distinguish objects, animals and even people from one another by their shapes. The simplest shape is a circle and things at a distance are perceived as dots. The dot when in motion becomes a line. The line when intersecting with itself becomes a shape. Even similar shapes have unique qualities and certainly the shape of all human beings are similar to one another but each individual is shaped differently from each other in both obvious and subtle ways.

We may think of ourselves as being shaped for life experience in functional or dysfunctional ways. We may be in excellent shape for an athletic activity and in poor shape for a love relationship. Our physical shape determines to a great degree how we perceive ourselves, how we feel about ourselves and even how other people receive and judge us. General body formations that people share have been linked to other human characteristics. Thin people, fat people, people of medium build may even share certain expressive qualities with others who have similar shapes.

We tend to use the word shape, which defines an entity, as also defining our overall condition. If a person says that he is in good shape, it may refer to the fact that he feels good rather than looks good. We sense that within our own minds and bodies the intangible qualities of ourselves may even have shapes of their own even though we are unable to perceive those shapes. We believe that the earth is round even though only the astronauts have actually seen it from a distance. The shape of time, space and of the universe are concepts that may never be proven to individual senses but the human need to accept and simplify experience may be reflected in our use of the word shape even when referring to such abstractions.

People who change their shape, i.e. fat people who lose weight or thin people who gain, are often changed in ways beyond their physical appearance. The shape of their world literally changes because of the differences in the ways in which they act upon and are perceived within their environment.

People have control over their own shapes to a great degree, given a responsive and flexible environment. Each individual must interact with the external world at the skin, the interface where body shape and space meet. The relationship between a person and space is interactive and determines change in both. The person acts upon the environment, takes from it and grows within it. In turn, the surrounding environment changes as well. For example, in a barren environment a person may grow thin. In a loveless environment a person may grow fat. Our shape is flexible; we adapt to heat, cold, wind and all weather by temporarily assuming body shapes which adjust to conditions. The fetus is shaped by and shapes the womb. Humankind shapes and is shaped by space. The environment can be tender and submissive or aggressive and hostile and so may alter its own shape as well as that of the person.

The creation of shapes in art is an interaction between the shape that is brought into existence and the shape of the space that is changed by its presence. The image which emerges is linked to the interaction each individual human has with space and the resultant shapes which are produced. In each experience, both in art as well as in life, we may ask whether the shapes that we create are healthy, functional, hostile, compatible, strong, vulnerable and in what way they can be altered to suit our needs.

Mind Over Matter

Don Seiden

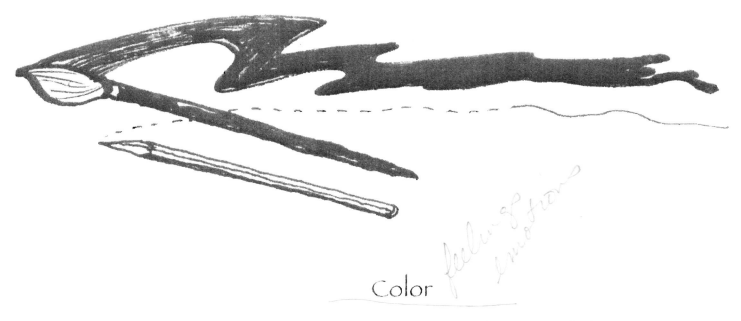

Color

Color, of all the elements, most closely resembles human feelings or emotion. Color in art may affect a physical as well as emotional response in the artist or audience. Color stimulates or depresses; excites or soothes, attracts or repels. Colors, in relationship with one another, can conflict, compliment, compete or cooperate and their connections arouse comparable feelings in the viewer. Because of the powerful impact that color has upon people, we often tend to interpret it's significance in isolation from other elements. This kind of interpretation reduces accuracy and limits meaning. Color must be associated with all other considerations and elements in order to gain a full understanding of the image.

Color affects and is affected by moods, atmosphere and quality of light. It is a pervasive element and one which has no boundaries so that the artist must limit and shape the color in his work. In this sense it can be used as a structural element. Shapes, for example can be built with color. Although colors have often historically been associated with psychological meanings, each individual must seek a personal response to color experiences and by doing so discover either universal or idio-syncratic meanings.

If line, shape, scale and motion are physical elements that describe visual images as if they possessed materiality or as if they were human, then color would generally define the affective, feeling qualities of the image and that quality of energy would then be communicated along with other more physical qualities.

Much like emotion, color can manifest various levels of intensity. It can be pure or mixed, saturated or diluted. Color can be flat or variable, blatant or subtle.

The artist/client who is unsure of his own emotional stability may react to the use of color in his art by refusing to use color, indiscriminately using it or by strictly separating one color from another as in a rainbow image. Mixing of colors and more subtle approaches require some degree of skill, confidence and self-awareness. The artist therapist may help a client to identify, become familiar with and to use color as an important art element in personal expression.

The colors of our skin, hair, clothing, eyes, the colors of our moods, feelings, the colors which may even describe experiences of life itself, are forces that communicate information about our selves. The word color, among other things, relates to pigment in art, to temperament and feelings in people, and to the quality of light in the environment. Art as therapy tends to focus attention on the use of color in art-making and how it relates to the emotional experience of the artist/client.

I think of color in relation to intensity of feeling people exhibit in their behavior. People express a wide range of behavior. If we think of this behavior in terms of color, clients/artists may then be described as exhibiting qualities which are hot or cold, dark or light, intense or subtle, transparent, vivid, receding, advancing and also as expressing relationships which may define conflict as well as harmony.

Color pigment tends to excite or calm us in its physiological effects on the nervous system. The "color" in behavior has the power to communicate and affect others by stimulating or depressing their moods. When a person, for example, is exhibiting "red" behavior and contacts an individual who is "blue" the result of that interaction may be a violet or purple dialogue. Violet, in one instance, is defined by Dr. Max Luscher, a color expert, as a "fusion between impulsive red and gentle blue which results in a mystic union in which hopefully, wishes are fulfilled" (Random House, *The Luscher Color Test*, 1969). Color, like behavior, is rarely pure. Profound despondency may be seen as a black mood, but it is often tinted with other colors, red, for example, which may represent an underlying vitality or power that is subdued by the negation of blackness. Yellow behavior which expresses a radiant, light, expansive mood may be tempered with subdued blue so that the expression begins to be a "green" communication. Individual cultures will define color symbols differently and thus therapists should be cautious in interpretation of those relationships.

Behavior may express "muddiness" that would imply too many colors or feelings mixing together there by losing their clarity. It may represent a monochromatic experience in which an individual communicates many shades of a specific emotional quality. A person may present or display inner battles represented by opposing colors which may be seen as being in conflict, i.e. red vs. green, yellow vs. purple, orange vs. blue. The quality and consistency may be related to a flow of warm or cool colors moving through reds and yellows or blues and greens.

Color relates to our awareness of light and dark. What does the night mean to us? The day? Tinting or shading a color by adding white or black shifts the visual and emotional impact of the color.

We are conscious of our own and perceive in others dark moods, light moods and the mixed or ambivalent feelings which are so common in human experience. As art therapists, the relationships that connect color and feeling are important ones both in the art created by our clients and the behaviors exhibited that may be altered through art therapy. A sensitive, trained eye sees color in nature that may not be readily apparent to others. A sensitive, trained eye detects behavior in people that may be subtle yet deeply meaningful. Color when used as an element in art may express strength, vitality, consistency and other positive qualities. Feelings in behavior may also reflect deeper, more consistent emotional strengths as well as the familiar, fleeting moods.

Don Seiden

The weather changes daily but the climate is consistent. We all possess certain basic and definitive "colors" in our persons, but we certainly may be capable of experiencing a full spectrum of colors in our daily expression.

In art therapy, color choices in art products are determined on a personal level by each artist/client. These color choices reflect attitudes toward color which have been conditioned by each individual's total life experience.

Mind Over Matter

Don Seiden

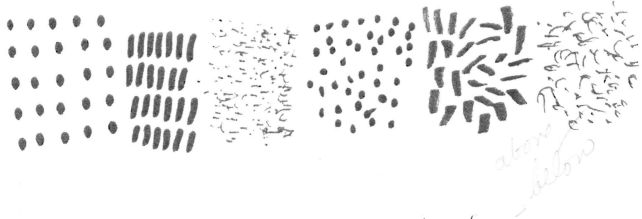

above
below

Experiencing Texture and Surface

The surface of a work of art possesses qualities which may stimulate our tactile sense. The work can be rough or smooth, flat, undulating or it may express other characteristics that attract or repel. The surface of an art object, like the surface of a person, communicates information about itself. The information may be designed to be seductive or hostile, crude or refined. It may be honest, open and may truly reflect the nature of the object or person or it may be a false image that conceals quite another entity.

Since the surface, like the clothing we wear, can reveal or hide the main substance of the object or person, we tend not to trust our sense of touch to tell us much about what exists below the surface. Touch, however, is profound in its ability to arouse and generate feelings, so that texture is an important element in art communication.

The tactile experience is intimately tied to our earliest memories of touching, holding and loving. Attitudes about touch may have early origins and may affect art making as well as human relationships. The making of art with particular concentration on texture can aid in re-stimulating positive feelings as well as opening up new patterns of perception.

The surface of an art object should be a natural outgrowth of a physical boundary that reflects honestly and accurately what lies underneath. It should not be something that hides the truth. If the object is to communicate its essential character, then the surface, like all other elements, should confirm that message.

Surfaces may reveal or conceal the form which lies beneath. The surface of a person may be expressed by the visual appearance of his skin and choice of clothing, by his questions and answers, interests, choices of work or play as well as through gesture, movement, emotional responses and other overt behavior. We constantly receive and send information to and from one another via surface communication. Sensory responses to stimuli are processed and judgments are made regarding the character and substance of the person who is being observed. Any further correspondence between people after initial surface introductions depend upon the intensity of their mutual desire to pursue more in depth involvement. In the natural environment we perceive surfaces that are seductive or repulsive. Surfaces that people exhibit are similar in that they can be rough, smooth, yielding, hard, soft, slick, sticky, hot, cold and, as a matter of fact, can be described with the same words that describe nonhuman surfaces. Our perceptions of one another are often influenced by the surfaces which are revealed to us upon initial contacts. Since first impressions can be so unreliable, in order to gain valid information about a person we must piece together the data received from various sense perceptions and create some unified, organized image. In art therapy this procedure takes place each time the therapist is introduced to a new patient. Often the personality as seen on the surface may be quite different from the initial art expression which is seen by the therapist. The art of the client/artist, of course, may also confirm or deny first impressions regarding that person.

Some of the surface experiences that influence our perception and judgment include nature of eye contact, body movement and gestures, clothing and concern about appearance, cleanliness and hygiene, speech, mannerisms, attentiveness, emotional expression, ideas and thoughts, sensory awareness, openness, aggressiveness and many other real as well as symbolic behaviors we experience in others.

Humans and animals, unlike plants, are not rooted into the earth. We live and move across the surface of the land. We are familiar with and aware of the broad, vast expanse of surface available to our wanderings. This natural connection to surfaces offers stimulating and adventurous experiences when we travel and are exposed to varieties of sensory encounters. Those encounters may stimulate rootless, frightened feelings or exciting, pleasurable emotions that seduce us. The same or similar qualities of seduction or apprehension occur in our experiences with people. The surface of a person may be the natural outgrowth of the structure from which it emerges or it may be a facade that hides an underlying truth. The surface may be rough or smooth, difficult or easy but it must be dealt with before any further depth involvement can begin to be created.

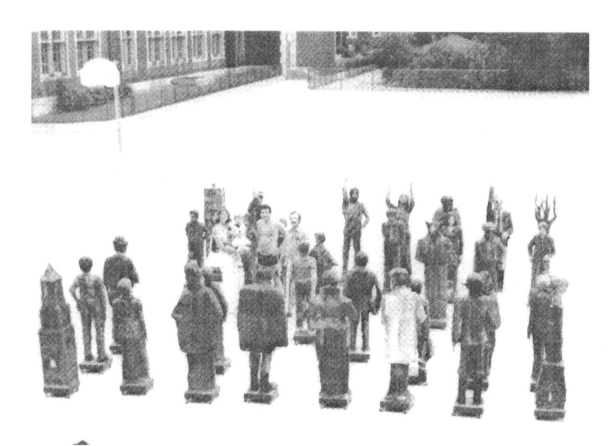

THE CHESS SET — Metal armatures for each figure are wrapped by screening. A resin is applied that is then painted. Each figure is placed into a concrete-filled aluminum box on casters that allow these large pieces to be moved around more easily.

Experiencing Size and Scale

The size of something conveys information about that thing, particularly when it is compared to the size of other things. When something is big or small we tend to read its size as a statement about its power, value, spatial needs, physical needs and even relative importance to other things.

In art therapy, clients/artists may communicate feelings of grandiosity, helplessness, power or lack of power through the scale of the work and the relative sizes of parts to one another. A tiny shape in a large space may seem to float, be unattached or appear helpless. The same small shape in a small space may appear quite different. Children live in a different spatial world than adults. Big children have power over small children. We are all influenced by the size of one another and these influences are reflected in art.

When an object is created which can be held in the hand, it allows the artist to feel powerful and controlling. When an artist creates a very large object, a different and more profound experience may result in that the artwork itself is now the source of awe and power. The artist may even feel dwarfed the art. Short people may compensate for their size by behaving aggressively while tall people may stoop in their desire to be unnoticed. The human body becomes the ultimate reference in judging response to the scale of an artwork. When people are asked to do a large drawing or painting one person may be unable to fill the space adequately and another may literally go off the page in the energy of creating images.

The symbolic potential of art relative to scale is important in art therapy. Size and scale can be elements which may help a person toward a more realistic self-appraisal, the development of a sense of power, and a clearer understanding of relationships. The positive or negative image of our physical selves is partially dependent on our actual size. It is also connected to the way in which our sizes are perceived by others. Size, the actual amount of space which we occupy, varies accordingly to the changes which take place in our growth, weight and even as to how we perceive our psychological space, that is, the space which we "need" in order to feel comfortable in our environment. Our imagination is stimulated by picturing ourselves as being giant or tiny in a world of normal scale. Our culture, our history perpetuates the idea that large is power and small is weakness. Although power and vulnerability certainly are not dependent on size or scale alone, much of our experience is affected by our perceptions of these elements.

The feeling that we have all experienced of being small must certainly have originated in early infancy and childhood. The dependency on bigger people and being overpowered by larger children is part of growing up also. Watch a child who studies an insect in his hands. There is a sense of power that permeates that experience. All of us have the capacity to feel big or small. As a matter of fact we are capable of experiencing the feelings of being small and large simultaneously. Physical obesity in a person may be experienced in terms of power. Large people may have small voices. Small people may have large voices.

Parts of the body may be larger in proportion to other parts. Behavior in a person is connected in some ways to the actual size as well as the perceived size of that individual. Some people tend to need more space than others. They feel more expansive. Some artists will work on grand scale projects, others will paint miniatures. All of us experience some flexibility in the scale of our lives. At times we feel closed in, smaller, and at other times we may feel as if we are being touched by others when they merely enter the space which surrounds us. We are affected emotionally by our size, relationships, scale and proportion.

It is interesting to observe that accordingly to Rudolph Arnheim in his book *Art and Visual Perception*, (University of California Press, 1954) children begin to draw size relationships in their art in the simplest way possible, that is, undifferentiated sizes of the various components of a picture. Things begin as equal in art and then as the need for differentiation arises the elements take on different sizes.

The reasons for various size relationships in art therapy products may be linked to factors like the relative importance of the various subjects, the distances represented, emotional or symbolic concerns and attempts to reproduce accurate physical size and related spatial relationships.

Mind Over Matter

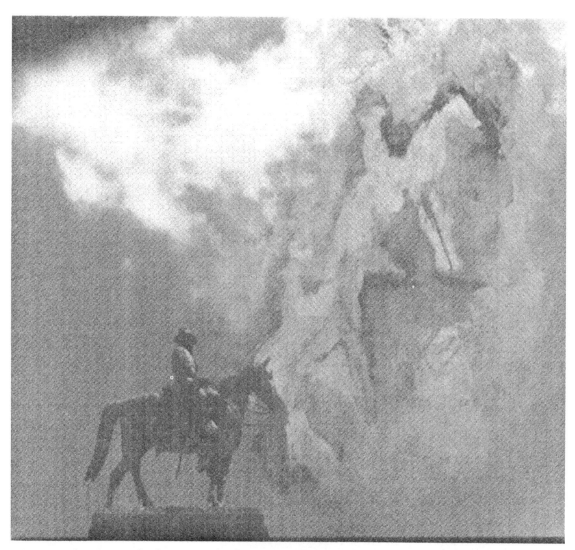

LOSS OF HEROES — The horses and riders are painted on the photo and then rephotographed and printed.

Don Seiden

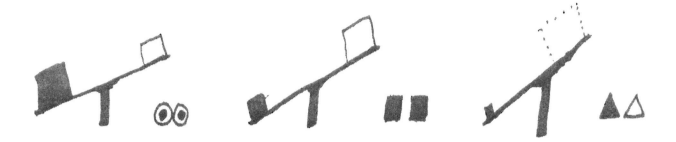

The Experience of Balance

To be in balance is to be stable, in control and secure. To be off balance is to be unstable, vulnerable and confused. Balance is a quality in art which refers to the relationship between forces which push or pull in one or another direction and the natural movement toward equilibrium. This relationship is a familiar one in art therapy since the clients/artists with whom we work are people who often are out of balance, in various states of tension and are seeking equilibrium. Art therapy provides an activity that deals with balance as part of the process of creating art. The various possibilities for achieving either balance or tension can be explored in the production of art which can then be further interpreted and studied as means for achieving desired goals in life experience.

Balance in art can be accomplished in a variety of ways from the symmetrical design where everything on one side is repeated on the other side, as in an ink blot, to the organization wherein equal but opposite forces offset one another. This correspondence of parts leads one to observe that nature seems pulled toward symmetry but living form seems relatively asymmetric and the human body itself is the most intimate example. Formal, symetrical balance can suggest stability or may seem lifeless; assymetrical balance brings with it a lively dynamic. The other extreme of balance, when equal but opposite forces are in balance, can be symbolized in a variety of images. A small but heavy object can balance a light but large one. A weak and transparent color which covers a large space may be balanced by a dense and vivid color which fills a small space. In art therapy, the images which the artist/ client creates may represent various states of balance and imbalance. These states are open to change and many possibilities exist for exploration and definition. The art therapist is to aid the artist/client in achieving desirable goals in relation to balance and tension.

In attitudes that relate to mental health, the word balance may be connected to our perception of emotional stability. We tend to value qualities of consistency and evenness that allow us to communicate with one another over long periods of time with a minimum number of abrupt and unpredictable changes in emotional behavior. We tend to mistrust people who exhibit behavior which is unbalanced or erratic. To be off balance is to be out of control, to fall, to be vulnerable, to be pulled or pushed away from an existing state. Everyone at times experiences a loss of stability. It happens physically when we trip or fall. It happens emotionally when we lose our temper, "fall" in love, or alter our sensory perception in unfamiliar ways. Some people, however, become unbalanced in ways that are profound and may be unable to regain balance in their behavior without help from others. This condition of helplessness that may be experienced in an unbalanced state implies a need to regain equilibrium through various means. The intervention of other people who seek to help compensate or reinstate balance may be important since an individual who is off balance is often unable to reinstate balance alone.

Symmetry defines a state of regularity and balance. It also implies a duality in which both sides are equal. As humans we experience both conscious and unconscious forces that direct our behavior, we are aware of the quiescent state of equilibrium when the equality or pressure from within and without are balanced. If this state, which may be seen as symmetrical, continues for long periods of time we may experience boredom due to a lack of tensions or, in some cases, a sense of awareness may occur that may be defined as mystical or profound. Balance in our moods and affective behavior may be cyclical. People may experience violent change in emotional stability from exuberant to melancholy in short periods of time. Violent and angry outbursts may occur in people suddenly and without apparent cause. Feelings which are normally flowing may be either blocked for various reasons and tend to create pressure or they may be stimulated and churned up to create turbulence. In addition, we also may be at the mercy of unknown forces which constantly change our state of balance. Permanent emotional balance is probably a fiction. We humans, reflect nature in that we seek equilibrium and rarely find it. Like walking, balance is an experience of falling and picking ourselves up again.

To be emotionally balanced then is to be in a state of relative rather than absolute equilibrium where the opposing forces are always attempting to equalize and when the push gets stronger, the pull resists with more force. The size, pressure and intensity of inner and outer powers vary and each experience brings its own forces into conflict. Normal life experience is a state of tension that seeks to be in balance. Only when forces are so powerful as to almost overcome the opposition do we recognize a state of imbalance. When a state of no conflict exists for a relatively long period of time, we describe that state as peaceful. Perfect balance in art as well as in life would require the impossible, a state of perfection and equal order created out of imperfect and un-equal parts that exist in harmony and conflict and create the tensions in their conflict which are the energy of life activity as well as the peace which is the product of equilibrium. Seeking the perfect, the impossible dream, however, is the work of art.

Don Seiden

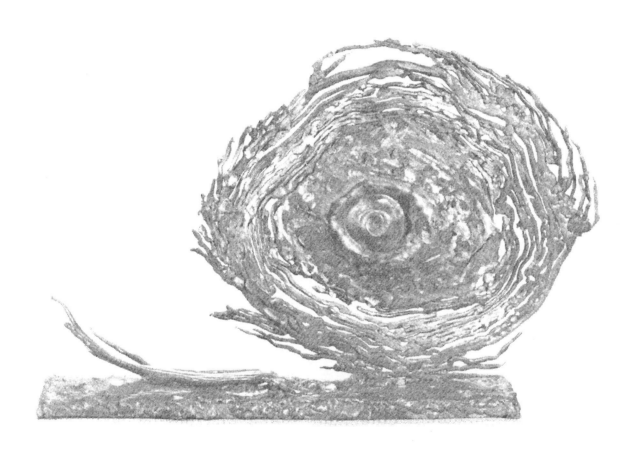

SEAFORM — Welded bronze rods.

Don Seiden

The Experience of Motion

Movement may be expressed in art both as symbol and as fact. A painting, although still and silent can express the feeling of motion while a sculpture may actually have moving parts. Dance and motion pictures rely on movement to communicate. Our eyes are immediately attentive to movement, particularly when other objects remain still. Motion, like other art elements, gives us information about the thing that moves. In the movement of others we sense power, weakness, danger, sickness, health, peace, relaxation, tension and other qualities that tend to define the function and state of the thing being observed. Humans and animals rely on movement for survival. Movement is in some ways a defining feature of life; in death there is no motion.

The process of making art involves movement and the art product communicates the nature and quality of the motion that created it. Since art therapy often elicits unconscious expression, the motion expressed in art may be the same as, or opposite of, the personal body movement that the artist expresses in daily life. The inner feelings of a lethargic, non-moving individual may be swirling and powerful and the art may express that energy or it may reflect a sence of apparent apathy. The exuberance of a person experiencing a flood of energy may be reflected in art but the possibility also exists that the unconscious self may be in a frozen state and that condition may also be reflected in the work.

Movement is a major expression in animal and human experience. The way that an animal moves, for example, describes its life-sustaining connection to space. Animals exhibit movement patterns that illustrate how they hunt, trap or chase prey. Some animals lumber, some flow, and some are abrupt. People in their movement also communicate a wealth of personal information regarding their own life-sustaining patterns. Our individual styles of all of our available body movements combine to describe a person who is confident, aggressive, rhythmic, afraid, clumsy or dull.

In art therapy we see art products which also reflect various symbolic or actual movements. The artists/clients themselves, in their own body motion express a variety of states. Individuals in emotional crisis can demonstrate changes in movement styles. In such a state they may walk stiffly or with great effort. They may pace swiftly back and forth in intense concentration or wander aimlessly in circles. Their bodily movement might describe ritualistic motions or exaggerate normal movement. All of these and other types of familiar motion attitudes are seen in mental health settings. Exaggerated movement may be a sign of emotional or physical injury. The struggle to regain normal movement that a wounded animal experiences has its counterpart in the loss or change of mobility which patients often encounter. This profound alteration in what each individual considers to be normal movement characterizes the degree and maybe the quality of emotional or physical injury sustained in person. If normal motion is blocked, inhibited or destroyed, a person has lost an important sense of self or identity. We tend to recognize ourselves in great part through our natural rhythms and motion. When these rhythms are changed, the changes affect our ability to synthesize experience, to be effective in confronting the environment and may produce a sense of awkwardness that inhibits our ability to coexist with others.

Body movement (exercise, dance and athletic activity as well as symbolic experiences in visual art) can be aimed at helping individuals regain normal locomotion and to integrate sensory experience in ways that aid in therapeutic goals of regaining identity, confidence, esteem and in eliminating undesirable ritualistic behavior which does not represent normal, easy locomotion.

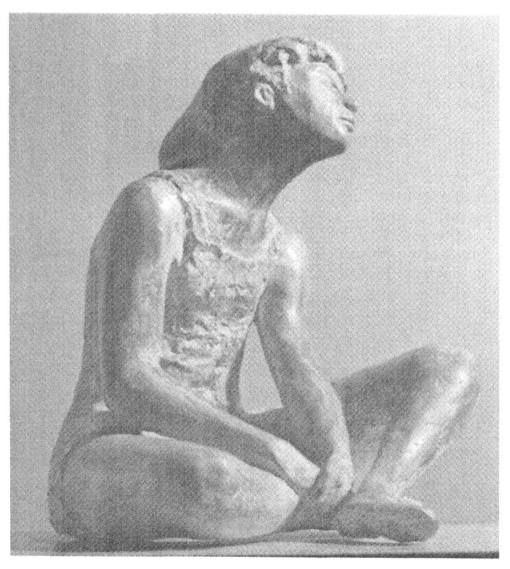

JUDY — Originally modelled in clay, then cast in plaster.

Don Seiden

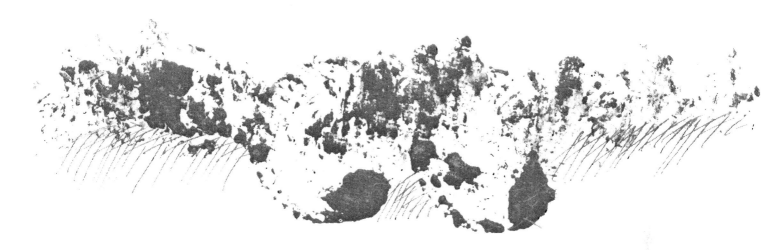

The Evidence of Experience

Art is the document, the evidence of experience. The object that commemorates an experience is still a THING. It is inanimate, not alive. Even a live performance can be recorded, photographed, filmed, or saved in a form other than the ephemeral moment of its presentation to a live audience. The preservation of life experience in the object is a magical thing. The stone sculpture speaks. The painting looks at me. The movie carries me through time and space. The use of symbols, those things that stand for other things, are the vehicle through which we can capture the past, the future and the present moment. We have explored various ways in which we can enter the art forms we encounter. We have discussed the elements of construction, the mechanics of forming, and inherent messages in a variety of media and materials in our world. Art is created by people and people communicate through symbols. The materials and the media live through the metaphor.

Mind Over Matter

Don Seiden

a Quick Reference
to Media and Behavioral Metaphors

ART & TECHNOLOGY — Video, Film, Photo and Computer Art are tools which offer the user a power and control over making things that is fast and accurate. They reflect contemporary life and give the artist feelings of mastery and status.

CARVING — Meeting resistant material and reaching the inner core of substance can empower the artist.

CASTING — Making and pouring molds suggests reproduction and continuation. The metaphoric change from a negative to a positive form is optimistic.

COLLAGE & MONTAGE — Securing a variety of materials permanently to a surface reflects a commitment to relationships, making the ordinary into something special and bringing diversity into unity.

CONSTRUCTION — Building by making step by step connections aids in achieving balance and control. Temporary and permanent connections can be achieved.

DESIGN — Planning ahead aids in problem solving ability, testing ideas and making judgments.

DRAWING — The making of marks on a surface is an immediate and intimate action. It confirms identity, as in "making your mark".

FIBER & FABRIC — Weaving and tying exhibit a "bringing together" (cohesive?) type of behavior that can be repetitive and familiar.

MODELING — Plasticity of material suggests easy manipulation, control in shaping and early tactile experience. Water based clay can be made permanent by kiln firing which raises the object in value and thus relates to self esteem

PAINTING — Color is often associated with feeling and is usually observed in painting. Flow, control-release, warm-cool, bold-passive. . . are some qualities that may be activated in painting.

PERFORMANCE ARTS — The variety of senses activated and the immediacy of response can be energizing and transforming.

PRINTMAKING — Reproduction of a print suggests continuity and the ability to replicate experience.

SCRAP & FOUND OBJECTS — The old and used can be viewed as valuable. The collecting brings a sense of security.